Medicinal Plants and Their Role in Preventive Care

Table of Contents

1. Introduction to Medicinal Plants

1.1. Definition and Historical Context

Medicinal plants have long been defined as those plant species that possess therapeutic properties that can aid in healing and maintaining health. Their relevance stretches well beyond just simple definitions; they have served as the backbone of numerous traditional healthcare systems around the globe. Many of these plants contain compounds that can alleviate symptoms, combat diseases, or support overall wellbeing. In various cultures, these plants have been integrated into daily life, making their study essential for understanding how they fit into both historical practices and modern applications.

Ancient civilizations have recognized the power of medicinal plants and have utilized them for therapeutic purposes for thousands of years. The Egyptians, for instance, relied on plants like garlic and myrrh, integrating them into their health systems for both physical ailments and spiritual practices. Ancient Chinese medicine, with its focus on balance and harmony, employed a wide variety of herbs and plants, emphasizing the holistic approach to healing. The Greeks also documented the use of plants in healing through the writings of Hippocrates, who is often referred to as the father of medicine, highlighting the significant role these plants played in early medical practices. Understanding these historical contexts enriches your knowledge of how medicinal plants have shaped healthcare throughout the ages.

As you delve into the world of medicinal plants, consider starting your own exploration by researching a local plant that has been traditionally used for medicinal purposes in your area. This practical tip not only deepens your understanding of the relationship between plants and health but also connects you to the historical practices that have been passed down through generations.

1.2. Importance in Traditional Medicine

Medicinal plants have played a crucial role in traditional healing systems across the globe. From ancient times, different cultures have relied on the healing properties of plants to treat a variety of ailments. Understanding the significance of these plants helps you appreciate their invaluable contributions to health and well-being. Each plant holds unique qualities that have been recognized and respected through generations, often forming the basis for holistic approaches to medicine that focus on treating the entire person rather than just symptoms. The rich knowledge of these herbal remedies comes from millennia of observation and practice, leading to methods that are often less invasive and more in tune with natural processes.

Examining case studies can reveal the effectiveness of these herbal practices in various cultures, showcasing vibrant traditions and approaches. For instance, in Ayurveda, the ancient system of medicine from India, herbs like turmeric and ashwagandha are celebrated for their healing benefits, ranging from anti-inflammatory properties to stress relief. Similarly, Traditional Chinese Medicine utilizes plants such as ginseng and ginger to enhance vitality and promote balance within the body. In each case, these practices demonstrate not only the effectiveness of the plants but also the deep cultural connections people have with nature. Observations from these cultures provide valuable insights into the importance of respecting and preserving traditional knowledge, as it continues to inform and enhance modern medicinal practices.

Implementing knowledge of medicinal plants into your own life can be both enriching and beneficial. Consider exploring local herbs and natural remedies that resonate with your health needs. Whether it's brewing a chamomile tea for relaxation or using eucalyptus oil for respiratory comfort, these simple practices bring a sense of connection to the long-standing traditions of healing that might inspire you to delve deeper into the world of herbal medicine.

1.3. Modern Research and Validation

Contemporary science increasingly explores the therapeutic uses of traditional medicinal plants, establishing a bridge between ancient practices and modern health solutions. By using advanced techniques, researchers now conduct rigorous studies to understand how these plants work on a molecular level. This validation process is crucial, as it not only supports traditional knowledge but also opens the door for integrating these natural remedies into mainstream medicine. For instance, plants like turmeric and ginger, long utilized in various cultures for their anti-inflammatory and antioxidant properties, are now being studied in clinical trials, yielding results that confirm their effectiveness in disease prevention and treatment.

Recent studies highlight significant findings that strengthen the case for traditional medicinal plants. For example, a surge in research has focused on the active compounds found in these plants, such as alkaloids, flavonoids, and tannins. A notable study published in a reputable journal demonstrated that extracts from the ashwagandha plant could reduce stress and anxiety, substantiating its historical use in Ayurvedic medicine. Similarly, research on echinacea has shown its ability to enhance immune response, making it a popular choice during cold and flu seasons. These findings not only provide scientific backing to traditional claims but also encourage further exploration into these natural resources for novel therapeutic applications.

It's important for you to stay informed about these developments as they shine a light on the potential benefits of incorporating medicinal plants into your lifestyle. Whether you're interested in herbal supplements or simply want to enhance your health naturally, diving into current research can empower you to make educated choices. Always remember to consult with healthcare professionals before starting any new treatment, as they can guide you in navigating the rich world of medicinal plants safely and effectively.

2. Understanding Phytochemicals

2.1. Types of Phytochemicals

Medicinal plants are rich in phytochemicals, which are natural compounds that play a significant role in promoting health. The major classes of phytochemicals found in these plants include flavonoids, alkaloids, terpenoids, and phenolic acids. Flavonoids, for example, are known for their antioxidant properties and are prevalent in fruits, vegetables, and herbs. Alkaloids, which include compounds like caffeine and morphine, often have pronounced physiological effects and can be beneficial in small doses. Terpenoids, found in essential oils, contribute to the aroma and flavor of plants and have been shown to have therapeutic effects ranging from anti-inflammatory to antimicrobial properties. Lastly, phenolic acids serve as powerful antioxidants that help combat oxidative stress in the body.

Understanding how these different phytochemicals contribute to the therapeutic benefits of plants is crucial. For instance, flavonoids not only enhance the flavors of food but also assist in preventing chronic diseases through their ability to reduce inflammation and improve vascular health. Alkaloids like quinine serve as crucial treatments for malaria, showcasing the direct medicinal applications of these compounds. Terpenoids, with their diverse range of biological activities, can aid in relaxation and stress reduction when used in aromatherapy. These compounds work synergistically within their plant sources, meaning that consuming the whole plant often provides a greater health benefit than isolating a single compound. By recognizing the therapeutic potentials of these phytochemicals, you can make informed choices about incorporating medicinal plants into your lifestyle.

Exploring local markets or herbal stores to find a variety of medicinal plants can be a rewarding way to experience their benefits firsthand. As you experiment with different herbs and plants, consider how their unique phytochemical profiles can enhance your well-being. Whether through teas, tinctures, or culinary uses, engaging with these natural substances can enrich your health journey.

2.2. Mechanisms of Action

Phytochemicals are compounds produced by plants that have significant effects on human physiology and disease pathways. You should know that these compounds interact with various biological processes in your body. For example, flavonoids, which are a type of phytochemical, possess antioxidant properties that can neutralize harmful free radicals. This action can potentially reduce oxidative stress, which plays a role in the development of chronic diseases such as cancer and cardiovascular disease. Similarly, certain phytochemicals can modulate inflammatory pathways, providing protection against inflammation-related illnesses. When you consume phytochemical-rich foods, these compounds engage with cellular pathways, influencing gene expression and promoting health benefits such as improved immunity or enhanced metabolic function.

Understanding the interaction between phytochemicals and your body systems can further highlight their potential health improvements. When these compounds enter your system, they may influence the digestive, immune, and even endocrine systems. For instance, some phytochemicals can enhance the absorption of nutrients and support gut health, leading to better digestion and overall well-being. Others might interact with receptors in your body that help regulate hormones, thereby influencing conditions like diabetes or hormone-related cancers. As you explore the world of medicinal plants, consider how the unique profiles of phytochemicals can enhance your health by supporting various body functions. Staying informed about these interactions allows you to make better dietary choices, potentially harnessing the therapeutic benefits that nature has to offer.

One practical tip for incorporating phytochemicals into your diet is to consume a colorful variety of fruits and vegetables. Each color often represents a different set of phytochemicals and nutrients, so including a rainbow of produce in your meals can optimize your intake of these beneficial compounds, helping to harness their full health potential.

2.3. Health Benefits and Risks

Common phytochemicals found in plants offer various health benefits that can significantly enhance your well-being. These natural compounds, such as flavonoids, carotenoids, and glucosinolates, provide antioxidant properties that help protect your cells from damage caused by free radicals. For instance, flavonoids, often found in fruits like berries and citrus, can support heart health by improving blood flow and reducing inflammation. Carotenoids, which you get from carrots and leafy greens, play a key role in eye health, helping to reduce the risk of age-related macular degeneration. Additionally, certain phytochemicals can boost your immune system, enhance metabolic functions, and even have an anti-cancer effect. Research suggests that diets rich in these compounds can lower the risk of chronic diseases and promote longevity, making them a crucial part of your daily intake.

However, while phytochemicals are generally beneficial, there are potential risks and side effects associated with their consumption that you need to be aware of. For instance, some individuals may experience allergic reactions to specific phytochemicals, such as those found in certain fruits and vegetables. Additionally, excessive intake of certain supplements concentrated with these compounds could lead to toxicity or adverse reactions, particularly in sensitive individuals or when combined with medications. It's also noteworthy that while whole foods containing phytochemicals are usually safe, attempting to extract these compounds for concentrated use might not yield the same health benefits and can sometimes be harmful. As with any dietary changes, moderation is key, and paying attention to your body's response is essential.

To safely incorporate the benefits of phytochemicals into your lifestyle, consider focusing on consuming a variety of whole, unprocessed fruits, vegetables, herbs, and spices. Each plant has its unique profile of phytochemicals, and a diverse diet maximizes your intake of these beneficial compounds. Always consult with a healthcare professional before making significant changes to your diet, especially if you have health conditions or are taking medications. This proactive approach not only enhances your health but also allows you to enjoy the rich flavors and nutrients that nature has to offer.

3. Common Medicinal Plants and Their Uses

3.1. Aloe Vera: Healing Properties

Aloe Vera is well-known for its exceptional healing properties, especially in skin care. Its gel-like substance is packed with vitamins, minerals, and antioxidants, which help to soothe and heal various skin ailments. When applied topically, Aloe Vera can reduce inflammation, alleviate sunburn, and promote wound healing. The cooling sensation it provides can ease discomfort associated with minor burns and irritations. Moreover, it helps to hydrate the skin without leaving it greasy, making it ideal for all skin types. This remarkable plant stimulates the production of collagen, supporting the skin's natural elasticity and reducing the appearance of fine lines and aging. Research shows that regular use of Aloe Vera can lead to healthier skin by maintaining its moisture balance and providing essential nutrients.

To utilize Aloe Vera for various health concerns, you can start by extracting the gel from its leaves. This gel can be used directly on the skin or mixed with other natural ingredients for enhanced benefits. For digestive health, consider consuming Aloe Vera juice, which helps soothe the digestive system and may alleviate symptoms of constipation. You can also explore using Aloe Vera as a remedy for acne by applying the gel on affected areas. Its antibacterial properties help fight the bacteria that cause acne while reducing redness and scarring. For those experiencing inflammation or joint pain, Aloe Vera can be applied topically or ingested to provide relief. Remember to do a patch test before applying it extensively to avoid any allergic reactions.

Always ensure that the Aloe Vera you use is fresh and preferably organic, as this maximizes its effectiveness and safety. To make the most of its healing capabilities, consider incorporating Aloe Vera into your daily routine, whether in skincare regimens or natural health drinks. This versatile plant not only enhances overall wellness but also serves as a valuable addition to your medicinal plant collection.

3.2. Turmeric: Anti-inflammatory Benefits

Turmeric, a vibrant yellow spice commonly used in cooking, is renowned for its numerous health benefits, primarily due to its active compound, curcumin. Curcumin is a powerful anti-inflammatory agent, making turmeric a staple in both traditional and modern medicine. Inflammation is a natural response by the body, but chronic inflammation can lead to various diseases, including arthritis, heart disease, and even cancer. By incorporating turmeric into your diet, you may help reduce inflammation, supporting your overall health. The benefits of curcumin in managing inflammation are not just anecdotal; many studies have highlighted its efficacy. For instance, research has shown that curcumin can block the molecules that play a significant role in the inflammatory process. This means that by consuming turmeric regularly, you can bolster your body's defenses against inflammation-related ailments.

Many scientific investigations have examined turmeric's impact on chronic diseases. For example, numerous studies support the use of curcumin in treating arthritis, as it can significantly reduce joint pain and swelling. In patients with inflammatory bowel disease, curcumin has been associated with improved symptoms and lower disease activity. Additionally, there is growing evidence that curcumin may aid in managing metabolic syndrome, which encompasses various conditions linked to inflammation, such as obesity and insulin resistance. By integrating turmeric into your health regimen, you may actively participate in your chronic disease management. The remarkable anti-inflammatory properties of turmeric suggest that your kitchen can be your first line of defense against chronic conditions.

An excellent way to incorporate turmeric into your diet is by adding it to smoothies, teas, or even savory dishes. However, remember that curcumin is not easily absorbed by the body. To enhance its absorption, consider consuming it with black pepper, which contains piperine, a natural compound that improves curcumin bioavailability. You can also explore turmeric supplements, but always ensure they are of high quality. Taking simple steps today can lead to significant health benefits tomorrow.

3.3. Ginger: Digestive Aid

Ginger is renowned for its ability to aid digestion and alleviate nausea. The active compounds in ginger, particularly gingerol and shogaol, play a crucial role in this. These compounds stimulate the production of digestive enzymes, helping to break down food more efficiently. By enhancing gastric motility, ginger helps in moving food through the digestive tract, reducing the chances of bloating or discomfort. This is especially beneficial for individuals who experience slower digestion or who suffer from conditions like irritable bowel syndrome (IBS). Additionally, ginger has been shown to effectively combat nausea, whether it stems from motion sickness, morning sickness during pregnancy, or the side effects of chemotherapy. Its soothing properties make it a go-to remedy for anyone seeking relief from an upset stomach.

Ginger's versatility extends beyond its medicinal properties into the culinary realm. In the kitchen, it's a beloved spice that adds warmth and zest to a variety of dishes. To incorporate ginger into your meals, consider adding fresh ginger to stir-fries, soups, and marinades. It pairs exceptionally well with both sweet and savory flavors, enhancing dishes like pumpkin soup or gingerbread cookies.

Beyond its use in cooking, ginger can be infused in teas for a comforting beverage that aids digestion and provides a therapeutic experience. Additionally, ginger has made its way into health supplements, with options ranging from ginger capsules to powdered extracts, making it easy to reap its benefits in a convenient form. With its myriad of uses, ginger stands out not just as a flavorful addition to your diet but as a powerful tool for maintaining digestive health.

To maximize the digestive benefits of ginger, consider incorporating it regularly into your daily routine. Even a small amount, such as a slice of fresh ginger in your morning tea or a pinch of ground ginger in your oatmeal, can make a notable difference. Keep in mind that fresh ginger is often the most potent form, so try to use it over dried versions when possible. Remember that everyone's body responds differently, so listen to yours and find the amount and form of ginger that works best for you.

4. Cultivation of Medicinal Plants

4.1. Choosing the Right Environment

Identifying the ideal environmental conditions for successful cultivation of medicinal plants is essential for anyone interested in gardening or herbalism. Each plant has its unique preferences for soil type, moisture levels, and air circulation. Begin by selecting a location with well-draining soil that is rich in organic matter, as this enhances nutrient availability and promotes healthy root development. Observing the area's drainage patterns can also help, especially after rainfall. Plants like lavender thrive in drier soils, while others, such as wetland-loving marshmallow, require significantly more moisture. Understanding these nuances will guide you in creating an environment conducive to growth.

Climate plays a pivotal role in the growth of medicinal plants, and it varies significantly from one species to another. You must evaluate the average temperature range in your area and how it aligns with the requirements of the plants on your list. For instance, many traditional herbs like sage and thyme favor warm, sunny environments, while others, like peppermint, prefer a cooler climate with partial shade. Light is another critical factor. Assess how many hours of direct sunlight your chosen area receives each day. Most medicinal plants benefit from at least six hours of sunlight, but some may require protection from the harsh afternoon sun. Additionally, consider the space available for growth; certain plants can spread out and need ample room, while others can thrive in tighter spots. Understanding the specific light and space needs of each plant will help you design an effective garden layout that maximizes their growth potential.

Finally, taking the time to observe the changing seasons and how your garden responds can offer invaluable insights. Note how the light shifts and how moisture levels change with rainfall patterns. This will not only help you adjust your care regimen but also enhance your understanding of the intricate relationship between plant growth and environmental conditions. Remember, the right environment is not just about meeting the basic needs of your plants; it's about creating a vibrant ecosystem that nurtures them to flourish. A useful tip for anyone getting started is to consider companion planting, which can help improve nutrient uptake and pest resistance, ultimately fostering a healthier garden.

4.2. Soil and Nutritional Needs

Understanding the types of soil that are suitable for different medicinal plants is crucial for their successful growth. Various medicinal plants thrive in distinct soil types. For instance, plants like echinacea and milk thistle prefer sandy loam soil, which provides good drainage and aeration. On the other hand, herbs such as valerian and catnip flourish in more nutrient-rich clay or loamy soils. Always consider the pH level of the soil as well; many medicinal plants prefer a slightly acidic to neutral pH, typically around 6 to 7. Regularly testing your soil can help you determine its composition and pH, allowing you to make necessary amendments for optimal growth and health of your plants.

Providing essential nutrients for optimum plant growth involves using the right fertilizers at the right times. Plants need a balanced mix of nitrogen, phosphorus, and potassium, commonly referred to as N-P-K. Nitrogen encourages foliage growth, phosphorus promotes root and flower development, and potassium enhances overall plant resilience. Organic options like compost or well-rotted manure can enrich the soil naturally while ensuring the plants receive vital nutrients. Additionally, micronutrients such as magnesium, calcium, and sulfur are equally important and can be incorporated through various organic fertilizers, ensuring that your plants not only grow strong but also produce potent medicinal compounds.

Incorporating mulching practices can benefit both soil health and plant nutrition. Mulch acts as a protective layer, helping to retain moisture and suppress weed growth. As it breaks down, it also adds organic matter to the soil, enriching it with nutrients over time. Remember that regular monitoring of your plants and their growing environment will help you make timely interventions. A practical tip is to observe the color and vigor of your plants; yellowing leaves may indicate a nutrient deficiency, while lush, dark green foliage usually signifies adequate health. By being attentive to these signs, you can ensure the best conditions for your medicinal plants.

4.3. Pest Management and Organic Practices

When cultivating medicinal plants, maintaining their health is crucial, and organic pest management plays a pivotal role in this process. You can start by implementing integrated pest management (IPM) strategies, which focus on monitoring plants to identify potential pest issues early. Regular inspection helps you understand the pest life cycles and their natural predators. Encouraging beneficial insects, like ladybugs and lacewings, can naturally keep pest populations in check. Planting companion plants that repel pests or attract these beneficial insects creates a balanced ecosystem in your garden. Rotate crops periodically to disrupt pest cycles and reduce infestations, as many pests are attracted to specific plants. Additionally, utilizing physical barriers such as row covers, nets, or sticky traps can provide direct protection while minimizing chemical use.

Natural alternatives to synthetic chemicals have gained popularity among those interested in sustainable plant care. Options such as neem oil, which is derived from the seeds of the neem tree, effectively disrupt pests' life cycles without harming beneficial organisms. Soap sprays can also be instrumental against soft-bodied insects like aphids and spider mites. These solutions work by suffocating the pests, while the ingredients are biodegradable and safe for your plants. You might also explore diatomaceous earth, which is non-toxic and can deter a variety of insect pests by damaging their exoskeletons. Herbal concoctions made from garlic or hot pepper can serve as repellents when sprayed on affected plants. By experimenting and observing how your plants respond to these treatments, you gain valuable insight into effective pest management within an organic framework.

Remember, the goal is to create a healthy environment that supports your plants rather than relying on harsh chemicals. This approach not only benefits your garden but also contributes to a wider effort of sustainable agriculture. As you delve into organic practices, keep in mind that patience and observation are key. Each plant and pest interaction provides a lesson that enhances your understanding of this intricate relationship.

5. Harvesting and Processing Techniques

5.1. Sustainable Harvesting Methods

Understanding sustainable practices is crucial for ensuring the longevity of medicinal plant species. When you engage in harvesting, consider the ecological balance and the health of the ecosystem. Sustainable harvesting means taking only what you need and allowing the plants to continue thriving in their natural habitat. This involves recognizing the life cycles of these plants, such as flowering or seeding periods, so you can harvest at the right time without depleting their populations. Choose locations wisely, avoiding areas that are heavily trafficked or already stressed by other environmental factors. By adopting a mindful approach to gathering, you help preserve biodiversity and ensure that future generations can also benefit from these valuable medicinal resources.

Knowing the best times and methods for harvesting medicinal plants enhances their effectiveness and sustainability. Certain plants are best harvested during specific seasons or times of day. For example, many herbs have higher concentrations of active compounds in the early morning when their essential oils are at peak levels. It's important to familiarize yourself with the specific lifecycle of each plant you intend to harvest. Use gentle techniques such as cutting rather than pulling, which can damage root systems and hinder future growth. Employing proper tools and techniques not only ensures the health of the plants but also the quality of your harvest.

Always leave enough of the plant behind to promote regeneration. A general rule of thumb is to harvest no more than one-third of the plant at any given time. This practice allows the plant to recover and continue its life cycle. Additionally, consider planting a few seeds whenever you harvest to contribute to the population of that species in the wild. Engaging in such practices enriches your experience and contributes to the overall health of the environment, encouraging a sustainable relationship with nature. Remember, every small action you take can have a positive impact on the sustainability of medicinal plants.

5.2. Drying and Storage Practices

Understanding the significance of proper drying techniques is crucial for anyone seeking to preserve the active compounds found in medicinal plants. When you harvest herbs, the way you dry them can directly affect their potency and effectiveness. The primary goal of drying is to reduce moisture content, which hinders microbial growth and degradation of valuable compounds. Whether you opt for air drying, using a dehydrator, or applying low heat methods, maintaining the right temperature and airflow is essential. Over-drying can lead to the destruction of delicate oils and flavors, while inadequate drying may result in mold and decreased shelf life. Aim to create a controlled environment where herbs can dry evenly and thoroughly to capture the full spectrum of their benefits.

Effective storage methods play a vital role in maximizing the shelf life of your harvested herbs. Once dried, it is important to store your herbs in a way that protects them from light, heat, and moisture, as these factors can quickly diminish their quality. Consider using airtight glass jars or dark containers to shield them from exposure. Keeping your herbs in a cool, dark place ensures they retain their active constituents longer. Labeling each container with the name and date of harvest helps you keep track of freshness and potency. Remember that correctly stored herbs can retain their efficacy for up to a year or more, provided they are kept away from humidity and direct sunlight.

As you continue your journey with medicinal plants, always keep in mind that the care you take in drying and storage directly influences the benefits you can extract during use. A simple practice such as monitoring the conditions of your storage space can make a significant impact on the longevity of your herbs. Pay attention to temperature and humidity levels in your storage area, and adjust as necessary to maintain optimal conditions.

5.3. Extracting Active Ingredients

Understanding how to extract active compounds from medicinal plants is essential for harnessing their healing properties. Several methods exist, each with its advantages and suitable contexts. One popular technique is steeping dried plant material in a solvent like water or alcohol, a process called infusion. This method works well for herbs with high water solubility. For more robust extracts, decoction is often recommended, which involves boiling the plant parts to draw out the compounds effectively. Another common extraction technique is cold pressing, ideal for extracting essential oils from citrus peels or herbs. Additionally, more advanced methods such as steam distillation can provide very concentrated extracts, particularly useful in aromatherapy and holistic remedies. Always remember to choose the method that best suits the plant material you are working with and the desired results.

Once you have successfully extracted the active ingredients, preparing those extracts for use in remedies and formulations is your next step. You can start by ensuring your extracts are properly concentrated for effectiveness. For instance, tinctures, which are concentrated liquid extracts, can be created by soaking the plant material in alcohol for several weeks. This allows the beneficial compounds to dissolve, resulting in a potent solution that can be diluted for use. Similarly, glycerites are another option for those seeking an alcohol-free extract. The combination of glycerin and water serves to extract plant properties while providing a sweet taste, making it perfect for children. When creating your own herbal remedies, consider how the extract will be administered, be it through teas, capsules, or topical applications, and choose carriers or bases that enhance the healing properties of your extracts.

Experimenting with different extraction methods and formulations can lead to more personalized remedies tailored to your needs. Keep a journal to document your processes, observations, and results, as this will help you refine your techniques over time. Understanding basic principles of extraction, along with practice, will also allow you to expand your experimentation into lesser-known plants, potentially discovering unique healing combinations. When working with medicinal plants, always prioritize safety by consulting reliable resources and practicing standard herbal safety measures. Remember, the journey of herbal extraction is not only about achieving results but also appreciating the plant's power and the wisdom of nature.

6. The Role of Medicinal Herbs in Preventive Healthcare

6.1. Holistic Approaches to Health

The holistic philosophy behind using medicinal herbs is rooted in the belief that health is not merely the absence of disease but a balanced interaction of the body, mind, and spirit. When you embrace this perspective, you begin to recognize that each herb has its unique properties that go beyond simple physical benefits. For instance, herbs like chamomile are known not only for their soothing effects on the digestive system but also for their calming influence on the mind. This interconnectedness suggests that by using medicinal herbs, you are tapping into a natural way to nurture your overall well-being. Instead of isolating symptoms, holistic herbalism encourages you to consider the whole person, promoting a deeper understanding of how different herbs can impact your health on multiple levels.

Integrating herbs into your routine can significantly enhance your overall well-being. Whether you choose to brew a warm cup of herbal tea, add fresh herbs to your meals, or utilize herbal tinctures, each method offers unique benefits that contribute to a balanced lifestyle. For example, incorporating herbs such as ginger and turmeric can support your immune system and reduce inflammation, while herbs like lavender and lemon balm can help manage stress. By making these small adjustments to your daily practices, you're not only enriching your diet but also allowing your body to naturally align with its needs. It's about creating a lifestyle that honors the wisdom of nature and prioritizes your health as a holistic experience.

A practical tip for integrating medicinal herbs into your life is to start a small herb garden at home. This could be a windowsill or a backyard plot where you grow easily accessible herbs like basil, mint, and rosemary. Tending to your plants allows you to build a deeper connection with the healing properties of these herbs while ensuring you have fresh ingredients on hand. This simple act of gardening not only supports your health through the use of fresh herbs in cooking and brewing but also provides a calming and rewarding experience that nurtures your mind and spirit.

6.2. Role in Chronic Disease Prevention

Certain medicinal herbs have long been recognized for their potential to contribute to the prevention of chronic diseases. The use of these plants is rooted in traditional medicine practices across various cultures, and modern research increasingly supports their beneficial properties. For instance, garlic is known for its ability to support heart health by helping to lower blood pressure and cholesterol levels. Turmeric, with its active compound curcumin, has anti-inflammatory effects that may prevent the development of diseases such as arthritis and diabetes. Additionally, herbs like ginger and green tea have been linked to improved metabolic functions and better regulation of blood sugar levels. Incorporating these herbs into your diet can serve as a proactive approach to maintaining your health and preventing chronic issues.

The evidence supporting the use of herbs in managing lifestyle-related illnesses is growing, with numerous studies highlighting their efficacy. For example, research has shown that cinnamon can improve insulin sensitivity, making it a valuable addition for individuals managing type 2 diabetes. Another herb, ashwagandha, has demonstrated the ability to reduce stress and anxiety levels, which are crucial factors in the management of heart disease. Observational studies and clinical trials alike provide insights into how these herbs can modify pathways related to inflammation and oxidative stress, which are often at the heart of chronic conditions. By understanding and utilizing these herbs, you can play an active role in managing your health and mitigating the risks associated with lifestyle diseases.

To effectively incorporate these medicinal herbs into your daily routine, consider starting with simple additions to your meals. Adding fresh garlic to your cooking, sipping on green tea instead of sugary beverages, or using turmeric in soups and smoothies are all practical ways to enhance your health. Remember that consistency is key; regular use of these herbs can yield cumulative benefits over time, potentially protecting you from a range of chronic diseases. Pay attention to how these changes make you feel and always consult with a healthcare professional if you are considering significant dietary changes or have existing health conditions.

6.3. Incorporating Herbs into Daily Routine

Integrating herbs into your daily life can be both simple and rewarding. Start by identifying herbs that excite you or that you feel would benefit your health. Fresh herbs can be easy to incorporate into meals; for instance, adding basil to your pasta or rosemary to roasted vegetables can elevate your dishes. Consider keeping a small herb garden on your kitchen windowsill. Basil, mint, and cilantro can grow with minimal effort and provide fresh additions to your cooking. You can also blend herbs into smoothies or teas, creating flavorful and nutritious beverages. If you find it easier, you might opt for dried herbs instead, sprinkling them on salads or using them in marinades. The key is to make herbs a regular part of your cooking routine, ensuring that they become as common in your pantry as salt and pepper.

Making dietary changes to enhance the preventive effects of herbs can significantly boost your overall wellness. Eating a diet rich in fruits, vegetables, whole grains, and lean proteins paired with herbal remedies can create a powerful synergy. For example, turmeric mixed with pepper can increase its bioavailability, making it more effective. Similarly, pairing garlic with olive oil can also enhance its beneficial properties. Consider incorporating herbs known for their health benefits into your meals, like ginger for digestion or nettle for its anti-inflammatory effects. Focus on balance and variety; this not only makes your meals more interesting but also ensures you gain the maximum benefits from the herbs you use.

One practical tip to remember is to experiment with different combinations of herbs in your cooking. Don't be afraid to try new flavors and ideas. You might stumble upon a delicious combination that not only enhances your meal but also promotes better health. Keeping a small notebook of your favorite herb combinations can help you track what works well for you and inspire you to keep experimenting.

7. Regulatory and Ethical Considerations

7.1. Understanding Herbal Product Regulations

Familiarizing yourself with the regulations governing the sale and use of herbal products is essential for anyone interested in medicinal plants. These regulations can vary widely depending on the country and region. It is crucial to be aware of the laws that dictate what constitutes a herbal product. This includes understanding the classifications, such as dietary supplements or cosmetics, which can affect how products are marketed and sold. You should also look into licensing requirements for manufacturers and retailers of herbal goods, as compliance with safety standards is vital for protecting consumers and ensuring product quality. Familiarity with good manufacturing practices will serve you well, as it highlights the importance of adhering to health and safety guidelines that are designed to ensure the efficacy and safety of herbal remedies.

Navigating compliance for herbal remedies involves an understanding of various regulatory bodies, such as the Food and Drug Administration (FDA) in the United States or similar entities in other countries. These agencies often publish guidelines on labeling, claims, and the necessary pre-market notifications that may be required. It is important to be aware of what claims can legally be made about the benefits of herbal products. Misleading claims can result in penalties or product recalls. Therefore, remaining updated on changes in regulations and actively participating in industry groups can help you stay informed about compliance requirements. Additionally, seeking advice from professionals who specialize in herbal product regulation can be a proactive way to handle any complexities you might encounter.

Staying informed about herbal product regulations is not just a legal obligation; it is also a commitment to consumer safety and your own integrity as a practitioner or entrepreneur in the herbal space. Regularly reviewing authoritative sources, such as government websites, industry newsletters, and academic journals, can help you keep current with new developments. Embracing education around these regulations will enhance your credibility and support your mission to promote the safe and effective use of herbal remedies. A practical tip is to create a checklist for compliance, including key regulations and standards, which can serve as a handy reference while you navigate the complexities of herbal product regulation in your endeavors.

7.2. Ethical Sourcing and Sustainability

Understanding the importance of ethical sourcing in the medicinal plant industry is crucial for anyone interested in these valuable resources. Ethical sourcing ensures that the plants are harvested responsibly, protecting not only the environment but also the communities involved in their production. When you source medicinal plants ethically, you contribute to preserving biodiversity and promoting fair trade practices. This can lead to higher quality products, as plants grown under ethically sound practices are often more robust and potent. You also help to maintain the cultural heritage of indigenous peoples who have been using these plants for generations, ensuring they receive fair compensation for their knowledge and labor.

Examining case studies that highlight sustainable harvesting practices reveals how the medicinal plant industry can thrive without compromising the planet. One notable example is the traditional harvesting of ginseng in North America. By implementing regulated harvesting methods that promote regrowth, local harvesters have managed to sustain their livelihoods while keeping ginseng populations stable. Another case is the use of shade-grown techniques for collecting medicinal mushrooms in forested areas, allowing the ecosystem to remain intact. These practices not only ensure a continuous supply of medicinal plants but also enhance biodiversity and support local economies. Learning from these examples can inspire you to advocate for similar sustainable practices in other regions and contexts.

A practical tip for engaging with the medicinal plant industry is to always ask questions about the sourcing of products. When purchasing herbal remedies or supplements, inquire whether they are sourced ethically and sustainably. Look for certifications or labels that signify ethical practices, and support companies that prioritize environmental and social responsibility. By making informed choices in what you buy, you contribute to ethical sourcing and sustainability, helping to create a healthier planet for future generations.

7.3. Intellectual Property and Medicinal Plants

Understanding intellectual property rights in medicinal plant research can be quite complex. Intellectual property refers to the legal rights that creators have over their inventions and the expressions of their ideas. In the realm of medicinal plants, this could involve patents on specific plant extracts, trademarks for product branding, or copyrights on research methods. The challenge arises because many traditional uses of plants have been known for centuries, passed down through generations of indigenous communities. Thus, patenting a plant that has long been used by local populations raises ethical questions about ownership and benefits. Researchers must navigate international laws and the varying standards of what constitutes innovation, creating a landscape where the line between protection and appropriation is often blurred.

The impact of these rights on access and innovation in herbal medicine is significant. When a company secures a patent on a medicinal plant or its uses, access to that particular knowledge or product may become restricted, affecting researchers, practitioners, and those in need of herbal remedies. This might stifle innovation, as smaller entities or local practitioners may lack the resources to compete in the marketplace dominated by large corporations holding numerous patents. Consequently, this can slow down the development of new herbal medicines that could potentially benefit public health. Understanding these dynamics can empower you to advocate for balanced approaches that encourage both the protection of intellectual property and the promotion of accessibility and innovation in the field of herbal medicine.

Being aware of the implications of intellectual property rights can help you contribute meaningfully to discussions about the future of medicinal plants. When engaging in research or practical application of herbal medicine, consider how these issues might influence your work or the communities you serve. Awareness and advocacy for equitable practices can foster an environment where traditional knowledge is honored, and innovation flourishes. Always seek to collaborate with local communities and understand their contributions, as their knowledge is invaluable in the ongoing exploration of medicinal plants.

8. Cultural Perspectives on Medicinal Plants

8.1. Traditional Practices Across Cultures

Across the world, traditions involving medicinal plants showcase the rich diversity of cultures and their unique approaches to healing. In many societies, plants have long been valued not only for their physical healing properties but also for the spiritual and cultural connections they embody. For instance, indigenous tribes in the Amazon rainforest have developed a complex understanding of local flora, using plants like ayahuasca in rituals to treat both physical ailments and spiritual imbalances. Similarly, Traditional Chinese Medicine employs herbs such as ginseng and ginger, which are believed to restore balance within the body according to concepts like yin and yang. You can find that these practices often involve deep respect for nature, highlighting the importance of maintaining harmony between the body and the environment.

Cultural beliefs significantly influence how herbs are perceived and utilized in healing practices. In many cultures, certain plants are surrounded by myths and stories that elevate their status and enhance their healing power. For example, in Ayurvedic medicine, the sacred basil, known as tulsi, is not only seen as a medicinal herb but is also revered spiritually, believed to offer protection and purify the environment. This intertwining of spirituality and healing is common, demonstrating how cultural narratives shape the ways in which plants are integrated into health practices. Understanding these cultural lenses can enrich your perspective as you explore the fascinating world of medicinal plants. To further appreciate these traditions, consider researching local herbalists in your area who can offer insight into regional practices and the cultural significance of various herbs.

8.2. Integrating Indigenous Knowledge

Indigenous knowledge plays a crucial role in understanding medicinal plants. For thousands of years, indigenous peoples have cultivated a profound relationship with the natural world, observing and documenting the healing properties of local flora. This knowledge is not just a collection of facts; it is intertwined with the spiritual and cultural practices of the communities. When you delve into the wisdom of indigenous practices, you uncover the intricate connections between plants, culture, and well-being. Understanding these relationships can enhance your appreciation for the medicinal plants you encounter, as you learn not only how these plants can treat ailments, but also the traditional contexts in which they are used. This layered understanding fosters a greater respect for both the plants and the cultures that have nurtured this knowledge.

Incorporating indigenous practices into modern herbal medicine can greatly enhance your approach to healing. Indigenous communities often utilize holistic methodologies, viewing health as a balance between the body, mind, and spirit. By learning from these practices, you can expand your toolkit for working with medicinal plants. For example, consider the traditional methods of preparation, such as the use of infusions, decoctions, or poultices, which may differ from modern extraction methods. You might also explore how cultural rituals and ancestral knowledge influence dosage and application, which can lead to more personalized and effective herbal remedies. Engaging with these practices not only enriches your understanding but also acknowledges the lived experiences and insights of indigenous peoples, paving the way for a more respectful and integrated approach to herbal medicine.

As you venture into the world of medicinal plants, integrating indigenous knowledge can transform your practice. One practical tip is to seek out local indigenous communities or herbalists who are willing to share their knowledge. This could involve participation in workshops, studying alongside traditional healers, or simply listening to their stories and experiences. By doing so, you can create a bridge between ancient wisdom and contemporary practices, fostering a deeper connection to the plant world and enhancing your own herbal journey.

8.3. Modern Adaptations in Therapy

Understanding how traditional therapies are adapting to modern health needs is essential for anyone interested in medicinal plants. Many of the remedies that have been used for centuries are being revisited and refined to address contemporary concerns such as stress management, chronic illnesses, and mental health. For instance, herbal treatments that were once solely used in cultural practices are now incorporated into clinical settings. This adaptation facilitates a more comprehensive approach to healing, combining the wisdom of ancient practices with current medical science. As you explore these integrations, consider how plants like ashwagandha for stress reduction or ginger for digestive health are gaining recognition in both holistic and conventional health practices.

Examples of successful integration of traditional and modern methods can be found in various therapeutic practices around the world. In many cases, practitioners blend herbal medicine with psychotherapy to create a well-rounded treatment approach. For instance, the use of chamomile not only serves as a soothing tea but is also recognized for its calming effects that can enhance cognitive therapy sessions. In addition, some healthcare providers employ acupuncture alongside herbal formulations to improve pain management and overall wellness. This integration showcases how traditional knowledge can enhance modern therapeutic practices, offering patients a richer array of treatment options that respect both the past and the present.

As you consider these modern adaptations, remember that the world of medicinal plants is vast and continually evolving. Engaging with both traditional and contemporary practices can provide deeper insights and more effective choices for health management. Always remember to consult with a knowledgeable practitioner when exploring herbal remedies, ensuring that you leverage their benefits safely and effectively.

9. Preparing Herbal Remedies at Home

9.1. Herbal Teas and Infusions

Herbal teas and infusions provide a delightful way to enjoy the healing properties of various plants. Each cup can embody a unique blend of flavors, aromas, and health benefits, making it a rewarding experience to explore this age-old tradition. To prepare herbal tea at home, begin by selecting your favorite dried herbs or fresh ingredients. For many, herbs like chamomile, peppermint, or ginger are good starting points. Measure about a tablespoon of dried herbs for each cup of water you intend to use. If you prefer fresh herbs, use a larger amount, typically around two tablespoons. Boil water and then allow it to cool slightly before pouring it over the herbs; this is especially important for delicate herbs. Let the mixture steep for five to ten minutes, depending on the strength you desire. After steeping, strain the herbs and enjoy your tea. You can sweeten it with honey or add a slice of lemon for additional flavor, enhancing both aroma and health benefits.

The terms tea, infusion, and decoction often create some confusion, as they describe different methods of extracting flavors and properties from plants. Herbal tea typically refers to the infusion of leaves, flowers, or fruits in hot water to extract flavor and nutrients. A simple infusion involves pouring hot water over the plant material and letting it steep, as you would with any herbal tea. On the other hand, decoctions are used for harder plant materials, like roots or bark. This method requires simmering the ingredients in water for up to 20 minutes, allowing for the extraction of more fibrous nutrients that would not yield their properties as easily in an infusion.

Understanding these differences can greatly enhance your herbal brewing skills. Experimenting with various herbs and infusion methods opens up a world of flavors and potential health benefits. As you become more familiar with the processes, you might even create your own unique blends that target specific wellness goals, such as improved digestion or relaxation. When experimenting, remember that while herbal teas can complement a healthy lifestyle, they should not replace medical advice or treatment. Keeping a journal of your herbal tea experiences could help you track what works best for you and refine your approach over time.

9.2. Tinctures and Extracts

Creating tinctures involves extracting the beneficial properties of herbs into a liquid form, typically using alcohol, vinegar, or glycerin. The process is simple yet effective, allowing you to harness the healing powers of various plants. Begin by selecting high-quality herbs that resonate with your intended purpose, whether for relaxation, immune support, or digestive health. After preparing the herbs, combine them with your chosen solvent in a glass jar, ensuring the plant material is fully submerged. Seal the jar and shake it gently to mix. Store it in a cool, dark place for several weeks, shaking it daily to encourage the extraction process. After the extraction period is complete, strain the mixture through a fine mesh or cheesecloth, and your tincture is ready. Tinctures offer numerous benefits, such as concentrated doses of herbal medicine, extended shelf life, and ease of use—making them an ideal choice for anyone interested in herbal remedies.

Understanding the various types of herbal extracts is key to selecting the right one for your needs. Extracts can be classified based on their preparation methods, concentration, and the solvent used. For example, fluid extracts are concentrated herbal solutions that contain a specific ratio of herb to solvent, providing a potent dosage. In contrast, powdered extracts involve drying the herb and grinding it into a fine powder, which can be used in capsules or mixed into foods. Furthermore, there are homemade options like decoctions and infusions that use water as a solvent, offering a gentler extraction method suitable for delicate herbs. Each type of extract has its unique properties and benefits, catering to different applications and preferences. By understanding these differences, you can make informed decisions about which extract will best suit your health goals.

As you explore tinctures and extracts, always remember that quality matters. Opt for organic herbs whenever possible, and pay attention to the sourcing of your alcohol or other solvents, as purity directly impacts the final product. Additionally, keep a journal of your creations, noting the herbs used, extraction times, and any effects observed after consumption. This practice not only enhances your understanding of herbal medicine but allows you to tailor remedies to your personal health journey.

9.3. Salves and Topical Applications

Making your own herbal salves for topical applications is both an art and a science. You can start by choosing your base oils, such as olive oil, coconut oil, or sweet almond oil, which are great for skin absorption. The next step involves selecting your herbs. Calendula, chamomile, and lavender are popular choices for their calming and healing properties. Start by infusing your chosen herbs into the oil. You can do this by gently heating the oil with the herbs in a double boiler for a few hours, ensuring the temperature remains low to preserve the herbs' beneficial properties. After that, strain the mixture to remove the plant material. You can then combine the infused oil with beeswax. The addition of beeswax will give your salve a thicker consistency and help it to stay on the skin longer. Typically, a ratio of one part beeswax to four parts infused oil is a good starting point. Melt the beeswax into the oil and pour your mixture into clean containers to cool and solidify.

The benefits of using herbal remedies for skin conditions are extensive and well-documented. Herbal salves can help soothe a variety of issues ranging from minor cuts, burns, and rashes to more chronic conditions like eczema or psoriasis. Many herbs possess antibacterial and antifungal properties, making them particularly effective in promoting healing and preventing infections. For instance, calendula is known for its anti-inflammatory qualities, making it ideal for irritated skin. Similarly, tea tree oil, when added to a salve, can provide powerful antiseptic benefits. By creating your own salves, you not only gain control over the ingredients, ensuring they are free from harsh chemicals, but you also engage in a holistic approach to self-care. This practice connects you with the healing properties of the natural world, enabling you to treat your skin with the same care and attention as you would any other aspect of your well-being.

When working with herbal remedies, it's crucial to conduct a patch test before applying any new salve to a larger area of the skin, especially if you have sensitive skin. A small amount on the inner wrist can help you gauge your skin's reaction. Remember, while herbal salves are highly beneficial, they are not replacements for professional medical advice or treatment. Always consult with a healthcare provider for persistent or severe skin issues. Incorporating herbal remedies into your daily routine can be a rewarding experience, so consider setting aside time each week to explore new herbs and create unique blends that cater to your skin's needs.

10. Safety and Contraindications

10.1. Identifying Allergic Reactions

Understanding how to identify potential allergic reactions to herbal remedies is crucial for anyone interested in using plants for health benefits. Allergies can arise from various components in herbs, such as proteins, essential oils, or even different processing methods. When you are trying a new herbal remedy, it's essential to start by researching the plant's properties and any known allergens associated with it. This initial step can help you understand what to look for as you begin to use these remedies. Awareness of your personal sensitivities is equally vital, as some individuals may have pre-existing allergies that can be exacerbated by certain herbs.

When you start experimenting with new herbs, pay close attention to any changes in how you feel or look. Signs of an allergic reaction can manifest in various ways, including skin rashes, itching, gastrointestinal discomfort, or respiratory issues. If you notice any unusual symptoms such as hives or swelling, particularly around your face and throat, it would be wise to stop using the herb immediately. Additionally, keep an eye out for less obvious signs such as sudden fatigue or changes in mood, which can sometimes accompany allergic responses. If you are aware of these symptoms, you can be more proactive in identifying and managing potential reactions, protecting your health as you explore the world of medicinal plants.

Always consider keeping a journal when trying new herbal remedies. Document your experiences, noting the herb used, the dosage, and any symptoms you might have felt. This practice not only helps in tracking allergic reactions but also builds a foundation of knowledge about what works best for your body. If an allergic reaction does occur, seek guidance from a healthcare professional and be prepared to share your notes. These records can be invaluable in assessing your responses and determining the best approach to safely enjoy the benefits of herbal remedies.

10.2. Interactions with Medications

Herbs are powerful tools in the realm of natural medicine, but when combined with conventional medications, they can lead to unexpected interactions. Understanding these herb-drug interactions is crucial to your health. For instance, St. John's Wort is known to reduce the effectiveness of certain antidepressants, birth control pills, and medications for HIV. This happens because St. John's Wort can speed up the metabolism of these drugs in the liver, potentially leading to lower drug levels in the bloodstream. Garlic, often praised for its heart health benefits, can also thin the blood, and when used in conjunction with anticoagulants like warfarin, it might increase the risk of bleeding. Recognizing these interactions is essential because they can have serious consequences, including diminished therapeutic effects or increased side effects. Always be aware of the herbs you are using and consider how they might interact with your prescribed medications.

Before you start using herbs alongside your medications, it is essential to consult with healthcare professionals. Doctors, pharmacists, or qualified herbalists can provide you with guidance tailored to your specific health situation. They can help assess the risks and benefits of combining herbal remedies with your current treatment plan. This consultation is especially important if you are pregnant, nursing, or have underlying health conditions that could be affected by these combinations. Healthcare providers can monitor your responses and adjust dosages as necessary to ensure efficacy and safety. They are invaluable resources capable of helping you navigate the complex landscape of herbal and conventional medicine.

As a practical tip, maintain a record of all the supplements and herbs you take. This detailed log can be very helpful during medical consultations, allowing providers to make informed choices about your treatment. Additionally, never hesitate to ask questions about any new herb or medication you are considering; being proactive about your health can help prevent adverse interactions.

10.3. General Guidelines for Use

Using medicinal herbs safely at home involves understanding their properties and respecting their potency. It is essential to learn about the specific herbs you plan to work with. This knowledge helps ensure that you are using them correctly and to your benefit. Start by researching each herb's uses, preparation methods, and potential side effects. Familiarize yourself with the proper dosages and how they can interact with any medications you might be taking. Keeping a journal of your experiences can also be beneficial, as it allows you to track how different herbs affect your body over time.

When it comes to dosing, it is crucial to start with small amounts of any medicinal herb. This approach allows your body to acclimate and helps you gauge how well you tolerate the herb's effects. Gradually increasing the dose can lead to a safer and more effective experience. For instance, if you are trying a new herbal tea or tincture, begin with a small serving and observe how your body reacts for a few days. If all goes well, you can slowly increase the amount, always paying attention to how you feel. This method of cautious exploration will maximize the benefits while minimizing any potential adverse effects.

Pay attention to your body's signals. If you experience any unexpected symptoms after consuming an herb, it's important to take a step back and reassess your use of it. Herbs can be powerful, and moderation is key. Remember, even though they are natural, they can still have potent effects. Always prioritize your well-being and stay informed about any herb you choose to explore.

11. The Future of Medicinal Plant Research

11.1. Emerging Trends in Pharmacognosy

As you explore the fascinating world of pharmacognosy, you will uncover cutting-edge trends in the study of medicinal plants and their compounds. Traditional uses of plants are being revitalized with modern research techniques, emphasizing the importance of these natural resources in contemporary medicine. Scientists are increasingly recognizing the therapeutic potentials locked within these plants, conducting extensive studies that unravel complex biochemical properties. New methodologies, such as metabolomics and phytochemistry, enable you to analyze plant compounds at an unprecedented scale, providing deeper insights into their functions and benefits. This integration of traditional knowledge with scientific inquiry is paving the path for innovative treatments derived from the rich biodiversity that our planet offers.

Your journey into herbal research is significantly shaped by modern technology. Advanced tools, such as high-throughput screening and bioinformatics, are becoming essential in identifying and validating the medicinal properties of herbs. These technologies allow researchers and students to evaluate thousands of plant extracts in a fraction of the time it would take with conventional techniques. The advent of artificial intelligence in data analysis further accelerates the understanding of plant compounds, making it easier to predict their effects and interactions. This combination of cutting-edge science and technology not only enhances the research process but also opens new avenues for sustainable drug development, ensuring that the future of herbal medicine is both promising and responsible.

Staying informed about these trends is crucial for anyone interested in the field of medicinal plants. Engaging with online communities, attending workshops, or even participating in field studies can enhance your understanding and appreciation of this ever-evolving discipline. Experimenting with herbal remedies and documenting your findings could contribute valuable insights to the broader conversation in pharmacognosy. Remember to approach your studies with curiosity and a willingness to learn, as the world of medicinal plants is full of surprises waiting to be discovered.

11.2. Impact of Biotechnology

Biotechnology is revolutionizing the way we cultivate medicinal plants, making the process not only more efficient but also more sustainable. Through advancements in tissue culture techniques, for example, you can produce a large number of identical plants in a controlled environment. This method reduces the time it takes to grow these plants from seeds and allows for the cultivation of species that might otherwise struggle in natural conditions. With the ability to manipulate environmental factors such as light, temperature, and nutrient supply, you're ensuring that these plants can develop their beneficial compounds without the stresses of unpredictable weather or pests.

In addition, biotechnology plays a significant role in understanding and enhancing the active components found in these plants. By utilizing molecular markers, scientists can identify specific traits that contribute to the medicinal properties of plants. This can lead to the selection of higher-yielding varieties that maintain or even enhance therapeutic efficacy. If you're keen on herbal remedies, knowing that biotechnology enables better cultivation and conservation of rare medicinal plants could inspire your gardening choices.

The implications of genetic engineering in herbal medicine are profound. Through genetic modification, it's possible to enhance the production of desired phytochemicals, leading to more potent herbal remedies. For instance, some researchers are working on plants that naturally produce higher levels of compounds like flavonoids or alkaloids, which have various medicinal benefits. However, this adds a layer of ethical consideration and requires careful regulation. As someone interested in medicinal plants, you can engage with these discussions, weighing the benefits of increased medicinal potency against potential ecological and health risks that genetic engineering might pose. Understanding these dynamics will not only enrich your knowledge but may also shape your perspectives on the future of herbal medicine.

Becoming familiar with the advances in biotechnology can inform your choices in the herbs you use and grow. Consider supporting local farms that adopt sustainable biotech methods, or if you're cultivating your own plants, explore how you can apply some of these innovative techniques in your own garden.

11.3. Integration with Conventional Medicine

Successful case studies reveal how herbal remedies can complement conventional medical treatments. For instance, in one notable case, a patient undergoing chemotherapy combined the treatment with herbal formulas known for their ability to support immune function and alleviate side effects such as nausea and fatigue. These herbs, like ginger and astragalus, not only helped in enhancing the patient's resilience but also improved their overall quality of life during the treatment process. Similarly, another case study involved using St. John's Wort alongside antidepressants. While careful monitoring was necessary due to potential interactions, many patients found significant relief from depressive symptoms when combining these approaches. Instances like these illustrate the potential for herbs to fill in the gaps where conventional medicine may fall short, providing a more holistic treatment experience.

The importance of collaboration between herbalists and healthcare practitioners cannot be overstated. When these two worlds come together, patients benefit greatly. A collaborative approach often leads to a more comprehensive understanding of a patient's health needs. For example, if a healthcare practitioner is aware of the herbal treatments a patient is using, they can offer better advice regarding possible interactions with prescribed medications. Furthermore, professional herbalists possess a wealth of knowledge about herbal pharmacology that can enhance conventional treatment plans. This partnership encourages an open dialogue, ensuring that all aspects of a patient's care are considered and more personalized solutions are crafted. Such teamwork ultimately fosters a safer and more effective healing environment for patients, allowing them to explore the most beneficial aspects of both conventional and herbal medicine.

To make the most of this integration, initiate conversations with your healthcare provider about any herbal treatments you are considering or currently using. Being transparent not only helps to avoid potential interactions but also allows your provider to consider how these treatments might be coordinated to enhance your overall health outcomes.

12. Case Studies on Efficacy

12.1. Success Stories of Herbal Treatments

Many remarkable success stories exist that showcase the transformative power of herbal treatments. Consider the story of a woman named Sarah, who struggled for years with chronic anxiety. Traditional medications often left her feeling detached and drowsy. In her quest for relief, she turned to herbal remedies like chamomile and passionflower. Over time, Sarah noticed substantial improvements in her mental well-being, experiencing fewer anxiety episodes and a greater sense of calm. Her journey inspired others to explore the natural alternatives available, highlighting the potential benefits of integrating herbal treatments into personal care routines.

The impact of herbal treatments can be profound, resonating across a variety of health conditions. For instance, the use of ginger has been shown to alleviate nausea, especially in pregnant women. Many expectant mothers have relied on ginger tea or ginger candies to manage morning sickness effectively. Another illustration can be found in the realm of inflammation. Individuals suffering from arthritis have reported significant relief through the regular intake of turmeric, which contains curcumin known for its anti-inflammatory properties. These narratives are powerful reminders of how nature's offerings can play a therapeutic role in healing practices.

As you explore the world of medicinal plants, consider documenting your own experiences or those of others. This personal archive can offer insights and encouragement for enhanced health outcomes. Experiment with different herbal treatments, ensuring to research each plant's uses and potential effects. Your journey with herbal medicine could uncover new paths to wellness, much like those inspiring stories you've learned about.

12.2. Clinical Trials and Findings

Significant clinical trials focusing on herbal treatments have brought valuable insights into the potential benefits and efficacy of various medicinal plants. For example, trials involving turmeric have shown promising results in reducing inflammation and alleviating symptoms of arthritis. Similarly, research on echinacea has explored its effectiveness in preventing colds and boosting the immune system. These studies often involve carefully designed methodologies that track participants over an extended period, providing clarity on how herbal treatments perform compared to conventional medicine.

The rigorous testing processes that validate herbal efficacy typically include randomized controlled trials, where participants are assigned to either the treatment group using the herbal remedy or a placebo group. This methodology helps to eliminate bias and ensures that any observed effects can be attributed to the treatment itself rather than external factors. Additionally, peer-reviewed studies play a critical role in evaluating herbal medicines, as researchers must present their findings to the scrutiny of other experts in the field. Such processes contribute to a growing body of evidence that supports the use of certain herbal treatments in clinical practice.

Understanding the significance of these trials can empower you as a student or a curious individual to make informed choices regarding herbal remedies. Always look for studies that are published in reputable journals and consider the sample size and methodology used, as these factors influence the reliability of the findings. When exploring herbal treatments, it's beneficial to remain updated on recent research, ensuring you are informed about the latest discoveries in the field of medicinal plants.

12.3. Analyzing Failures: What Went Wrong?

Case studies can provide valuable insights into the shortcomings of certain herbal treatments. One notable example is the use of St. John's Wort for depression. Although this herb has been popular, numerous studies have revealed inconsistent results regarding its efficacy. In some cases, patients reported minimal relief, while others experienced side effects that outweighed the benefits. Similarly, another case study highlighted the use of echinacea for colds. While it is often marketed as an immune booster, scientific evidence has shown that it may not significantly reduce the duration or severity of cold symptoms for everyone. These shortcomings illustrate the importance of rigorously testing herbal remedies across diverse populations and conditions to prevent misleading claims and ensure patient safety.

Understanding the factors that lead to the failure of herbal remedies is crucial for both practitioners and consumers. One significant issue is the variability in the quality of herbal products. The herbal market is largely unregulated, which means that potency, purity, and formulation can vary greatly between brands. Additionally, the lack of standardization in dosages can hinder therapeutic outcomes. Another factor involves individual differences in biology; each person's metabolism, genetics, and existing health conditions can affect how an herbal remedy works. Furthermore, the presence of other medications can lead to interactions that may diminish efficacy or cause adverse effects. All these variables highlight the complexity of herbal treatments and the need for informed decision-making.

When exploring herbal remedies, always research the specific product and its background. Look for studies that support claims and check for certifications on quality and safety. Engaging in conversations with knowledgeable health professionals can also guide your choices and enhance your understanding of how these treatments work within a broader context of holistic health.

13. Global Trade and Medicinal Plants

13.1. Economic Impact of Herbal Markets

The global herbal market significantly influences local economies, acting as a vital source of income for many communities. As the demand for natural remedies rises, local growers and suppliers of medicinal plants find increased opportunities for business expansion. This market not only provides jobs but also encourages sustainable agricultural practices. With communities cultivating herbs for local markets or exports, the economic boost can lead to enhanced infrastructure and improved living standards. Understanding the dynamics of this market can empower you to support local economies while exploring the benefits of herbal medicine.

The growth of herbal markets reflects a rising consumer demand for natural and holistic health solutions. People are increasingly seeking alternatives to conventional medicine, leading to expanded interest in products derived from medicinal plants. As awareness spreads about the benefits of herbs, businesses are responding by developing innovative products, ranging from teas and essential oils to supplements and skincare items. This surge in interest not only drives economic activity but also fosters a greater appreciation for traditional knowledge and practices surrounding herbal medicine. Staying informed about this growing trend allows you to engage with a movement that prioritizes wellness and sustainability, ultimately enriching your understanding of medicinal plants.

Consider becoming involved in local herbal markets or community-supported agriculture initiatives. By purchasing from local growers, you contribute to the local economy while gaining access to fresh, potent herbal products. This action not only benefits your health but also strengthens the bonds within your community and supports sustainable farming practices.

13.2. Trade Regulations and Challenges

Understanding the challenges associated with trade regulations for medicinal plants is essential for anyone interested in this field. The world of medicinal plants is complex, and numerous regulations govern how these plants can be harvested, traded, and used. One significant challenge you might face involves navigating the various legal requirements in different countries. Each country has its own set of laws aimed at protecting biodiversity, ensuring safety, and preserving traditional knowledge. You may encounter restrictions that limit the export of certain species, especially those deemed endangered or threatened. Additionally, maintaining the quality and authenticity of plant products poses another challenge. Counterfeit or adulterated products can slip into the market, undermining both safety and trust in herbal remedies.

International efforts to regulate the herbal trade have grown significantly in recent years due to its popularity. Various organizations, including the World Health Organization (WHO) and the Convention on Biological Diversity (CBD), are implementing frameworks aimed at promoting sustainable practices. These initiatives often focus on ensuring that trade does not harm local ecosystems while also protecting the rights of indigenous communities who have traditionally used these plants. Knowing about these international laws can equip you with the tools to engage responsibly and ethically in the herbal trade. Staying informed about treaties and agreements that affect the herbal market is key to ensuring compliance and fostering sustainable practices.

As you explore the world of medicinal plants, it is helpful to stay connected with local and international organizations that promote ethical trade practices. These groups often provide resources and updates that can keep you informed about changes in regulations and best practices. Engaging with communities involved in medicinal plant trade can deepen your understanding and help you navigate the complexities of trade regulations effectively.

13.3. Case Studies in Global Sourcing

Successful case studies in the global sourcing of medicinal plants provide valuable insights into the practice and its transformative potential. For instance, consider the case of turmeric, sourced primarily from India. This vibrant yellow spice is not just a culinary staple; it holds significant medicinal properties, including anti-inflammatory and antioxidant effects. Through global sourcing, companies established partnerships with local farmers, providing them with fair trade opportunities and ensuring sustainable harvesting practices. This not only increased the quality and quantity of medicinal turmeric available on a global scale but also empowered local communities economically by giving them a stable income and access to global markets.

The impact of global sourcing on local communities goes beyond economics. It enriches cultural knowledge and encourages the preservation of traditional practices. Take, for example, the sourcing of ginseng from rural areas in Korea and China. As these regions become more integrated into global supply chains, local farmers are motivated to preserve their ancient farming and harvesting techniques that have been passed down through generations. This not only sustains the unique characteristics of the medicinal plants but also fosters a sense of pride and purpose among the local community. The challenge lies in ensuring that these benefits reach all community members equitably, promoting social responsibility within the global marketplace.

By engaging with local farmers and understanding their needs, businesses can create a win-win situation. Knowledge sharing is essential; companies can offer training in sustainable practices, while local communities provide invaluable expertise in traditional harvesting methods. This symbiotic relationship enhances the overall integrity and sustainability of global sourcing practices. Cultivating these connections can lead to innovative approaches in the industry, ensuring that as you study medicinal plants, you also appreciate the intricate web of relationships that make their sourcing possible.

14. Personalizing Herbal Medicine

14.1. Tailoring Herbal Remedies to Individual Needs

Customizing herbal remedies is essential for achieving the best results in your health journey. Every person is unique, and so are their health needs. Factors such as age, gender, lifestyle, and pre-existing conditions can greatly influence how you respond to different herbs. For instance, someone with a mild anxiety problem may benefit from herbs like chamomile or lemon balm, while another person with more severe anxiety may require stronger adaptogens like ashwagandha or rhodiola. Recognizing these differences allows you to select herbs that are not only safe but also effective for your specific conditions.

Conducting a personal health assessment is a critical step in guiding your herb selection. Begin by evaluating your personal health history, current symptoms, and any medications you are taking. It can be helpful to keep a journal where you document your daily experiences and any health changes you notice over time. This will give you insights into which areas of your health need the most attention. Additionally, be mindful of how different herbs affect your body as some may interact with medications or worsen certain conditions. Consulting with a qualified herbalist or healthcare professional can further refine your choices, ensuring that the herbal remedies you choose harmonize with your unique body and its requirements.

Personalized herbal remedies can lead to more effective and satisfying health outcomes. Through understanding your body and its specific needs, you empower yourself to make informed decisions about the plants that will support your wellness. When you approach herbal medicine as a tailored experience rather than a one-size-fits-all solution, you embrace a holistic approach that fosters balance and healing. Start today by paying close attention to how various herbs

make you feel, and don't hesitate to experiment under guided
supervision to discover what truly works for you.

14.2. Understanding Body Types and Herbal Compatibility

Your body type can significantly influence how herbal medicines
work for you. Different body compositions, metabolism rates, and
energy levels mean that not all herbs will have the same effects on
everyone. For instance, some individuals may have a slower
metabolism that processes herbs differently, leading to either
extended benefits or slower responses. Knowing your body type
helps to identify which herbs will have a more potent impact,
ensuring that you receive the full benefits. For example, warm-
natured body types may find that cooling herbs, like peppermint,
enhance their wellness, while cooling body types might require
warming herbs like ginger to stimulate their systems. This
knowledge allows for a tailored approach to using herbal remedies
effectively.

Choosing the right herbs that align with your body type is essential
for optimizing their effects. A good starting point is to assess your
dominant traits: Are you more energetic or lethargic? Warm or cool?
Once you have identified your main characteristics, you can select
herbs that complement your body's needs. If you tend toward a
heavier, more grounded body type, lighter herbs such as dandelion or
chamomile may help balance your energy levels. Conversely, if you
are more airy and tend to feel scattered, grounding herbs like
ashwagandha can help stabilize your energy and bring focus.
Understanding this compatibility not only enhances the efficacy of
the herbs you select but also fosters a deeper connection with the
plant kingdom.

Taking time to observe how different herbs affect you personally can
lead to more meaningful results. Keep a journal detailing your
experiences with various herbal remedies, noting how they influence
your mood, energy levels, and overall well-being. Regular reflection
on this journey will help you recognize patterns and refine your
choices, creating a personalized approach to herbal medicine that

resonates with your unique body type. This practice can serve as a guide not just for improving health but also for building a lifelong relationship with the plants that can nurture and heal.

14.3. The Role of Consultation in Personalized Medicine

Consulting with herbal professionals can significantly enhance your journey in personalized care. These experts bring a wealth of knowledge and experience that can be tailored to your specific health needs. They can help you navigate the vast world of medicinal plants, guiding you toward the herbs that align with your unique constitution and health goals. Whether you are seeking remedies for stress, digestive issues, or immune support, a professional consultation ensures that you are not only choosing the right herbs but also using them safely and effectively. Personalized guidance can lead to more meaningful results, as herbal professionals can help you understand the nuances of how different plants interact with your body, potential side effects, and the most beneficial ways to incorporate these herbs into your daily routine.

Ongoing discussions with herbal professionals are equally important for successful use of herbal remedies. The world of herbal medicine is not static; it evolves as your body responds to different treatments. Regular check-ins allow for adjustments based on your experiences, which can lead to optimized results. It's an opportunity to share any changes in your condition or concerns that may arise. This collaborative approach fosters a deeper understanding of your body's responses and promotes trust between you and your herbalist. Engaging in continuous dialogue not only enhances your knowledge but also empowers you to take an active role in your health decision-making process.

Ultimately, integrating consultation and ongoing discussions into your approach to herbal medicine enriches your experience and outcomes. Prioritize relationships with herbal professionals who value your input and engage in a two-way conversation about your health journey. This engagement can illuminate new avenues for exploration in the realm of medicinal plants, ensuring that your path to wellness is both informed and responsive to the changes in your body. Take the initiative to ask questions and explore topics that resonate with you, making the most of your personalized care experience.

15. Resources for Further Exploration

15.1. Key Literature and Research Articles

Identifying key literature on medicinal plants is essential for anyone interested in the benefits and applications of herbal remedies. Prominent texts such as "The Green Pharmacy" by James Duke provide a comprehensive overview of various plants, their usage in traditional medicine, and scientific validation. Another significant work is "Medicinal Plants of the World" by Ben-Erik van Wyk, which serves as both a reference guide and a source of interesting anecdotes about plant history and cultural significance. Exploring these texts offers insight into phytochemistry and ethnobotany, allowing you to appreciate how different cultures have utilized these plants throughout history.

Research articles play a crucial role in enhancing our understanding of herbal medicine by presenting new findings, clinical trials, and reviews of existing studies. For instance, sources such as the Journal of Ethnopharmacology and Phytotherapy Research regularly publish peer-reviewed articles that dive deep into specific plants and their medicinal effects. Articles exploring the efficacy of turmeric in anti-inflammatory therapies or the use of ginseng for energy enhancement provide practical, research-backed insights that can significantly influence your perspective on each herb's potential. Engaging with these articles equips you with evidence-based knowledge that can inform your own practices or enhance your academic studies.

As you delve into these resources, consider keeping a personal journal to note interesting findings, potential applications for your studies or personal use, and reflections on how different cultures integrate these plants into their healing traditions. This approach will not only enhance your learning experience but also enable you to develop a deeper connection with the plant kingdom.

15.2. Online Communities and Forums

Discovering online communities where you can connect with others interested in medicinal plants can be an invaluable resource on your journey. Numerous platforms exist, each providing space for those passionate about herbal medicine and natural healing. Websites like Reddit host subreddits focused on herbalism and natural remedies, where you can engage in conversations, ask questions, and share experiences with fellow enthusiasts. Facebook groups dedicated to medicinal plants also offer a warm environment to exchange knowledge. These communities often feature members ranging from novices to seasoned experts, ensuring that you can find support and information regardless of your skill level. Engaging with these groups not only enhances your understanding but can also lead to friendships with like-minded individuals who share your passion for the healing properties of plants.

Forums specifically designed for discussion and knowledge sharing around medicinal plants play an equally important role in your learning journey. Websites such as the Herb Society of America's forum provide a structured space for in-depth discussions on topics like plant identification, cultivation methods, and therapeutic applications. These forums allow you to participate in ongoing discussions or start your own threads to get insight on a particular topic. Many of these platforms also feature experienced herbalists who regularly contribute, offering advice and sharing their personal experiences. Engaging with these knowledgeable members can dramatically deepen your understanding of medicinal plants and promote critical thinking about your own practices.

Participating actively in online communities and forums can not only enhance your knowledge but also provide you with access to a wealth of resources, including articles, research papers, and workshops offered by experienced practitioners. Consider sharing your own insights and experiences, as contributing to these discussions not only helps others but also reinforces your knowledge and understanding. This collaborative learning environment is one of the best ways to explore the intricacies of medicinal plants and become part of a vibrant community dedicated to health and wellness.

15.3. Workshops and Seminars on Medicinal Plants

Finding workshops and seminars that focus on herbal medicine can significantly deepen your understanding of medicinal plants. These events often bring together experts and enthusiasts who share insights into the use of various herbs, their properties, and their applications in healing practices. Many workshops offer lectures, demonstrations, and interactive sessions where you can learn about identifying plants in their natural habitats, preparing herbal remedies, and understanding the science behind their medicinal properties. Engaging with professionals in the field allows you to ask questions, clarify doubts, and receive guidance tailored to your interests.

Hands-on experiences are invaluable when it comes to learning about medicinal plants. Not only do they provide practical knowledge, but they also enhance your ability to recognize different species and understand their uses. By participating in activities like plant foraging, you can develop skills that are hard to acquire through books alone. This experiential learning reinforces your understanding, as you gain insights into the plants' growth habits, seasonal availability, and the best practices for sustainable harvesting. Whether you are learning to make tinctures, salves, or teas, the tactile nature of these workshops allows you to connect with the plants on a deeper level.

As you explore various workshops, consider looking for those that also emphasize local medicinal plants or traditional healing practices unique to your region. This not only enriches your knowledge but immerses you in the cultural context surrounding herbal medicine. One practical tip for maximizing your experience is to network during these events. Connect with fellow attendees, share experiences, and exchange contact information. Building a community of like-minded individuals can enhance your learning journey and provide ongoing support as you delve deeper into the world of medicinal plants.

About the Author

Oludare Ogunde holds a degree in botany from the University of Lagos, Nigeria, where he developed a profound understanding of plant life and its numerous applications. His expertise includes:

- In-depth knowledge of medicinal plants

- Specialization in pharmacognosy

- Practical experience with natural remedies and healing properties of plants

Currently residing in Richmond, Virginia, U.S.A, Oludare draws from his rich cultural heritage and scientific background to explore the intricate relationships between humans and plants. His passion for botany and its medicinal aspects is reflected in his writings, where he aims to educate and inspire others to embrace the healing power of nature.

9 798346 106647